How to Get Rid of a Bruise

By

Kimberly Peters

For

26 Ways.com

Disclaimer

We are not doctors and we have no medical training. Therefore this publication is not intended to provide medical guidance, diagnosis or specific medical treatment. No part of this book was designed or intended to be used as a treatment program for any specific situation. Only a qualified medical professional can determine the proper treatment or course of action. We suggest you consult with your physician before taking any action. Since everyone is different and every situation is different there is no one cookie cutter approach or solution for every situation. The writers, publishers and sellers of this book assume no responsibility for the use or application of any or all parts of this book. The reader assumes total responsibility for deciding the suitability of any part of this book for their personal situation. Again, we suggest consulting with your physician on all medical treatment matters.

Contents

What is a Bruise?

In order to understand how to treat something, we first need to understand what it is. So let's begin with an explanation of what a bruise is.

A bruise is the result of tearing or rupturing of small blood vessels under our skin. They are usually caused by a bump, fall or other impact that produces a trauma to the area. Most of the time bruises are more of an inconvenience rather than a serious medical condition especially when they are located in areas that are visible to others.

But there may be times when bruises are just a symptom of a medical issue that may need medical attention. Though an impact or trauma is usually required to form a bruise, sometimes health issues or problems might make us more susceptible to bruising or result in more serious bruising than normal. The bruises may look exactly the same as a bruise caused by a fall or impact but they were caused by other factors.

Another term for a bruise is called a contusion. Bruises usually start out as a dark shade of purple and will get lighter and turn yellowish as they heal and the blood is absorbed into the body through the healing process. Eventually, all of the old blood will be absorbed by the body and all traces of the bruise will disappear,

Are Bruises Serious?

While most bruises are common and will take care of themselves without any action on our part, sometimes a bruise is merely a symptom of something more serious going on within our bodies.

If a bruise doesn't seem to heal or constantly gets darker and larger, this might mean that the bleeding has not stopped for some reason. When this occurs you should seriously consider getting medical attention if even just to get some peace of mind. If you start to run a fever, or if the area around the bruise should continue to swell or get hard, this could signal the presence of a hematoma which is a pool of blood under the skin. These may have to be drained by a doctor.

As far as medical attention is required keep in mind that bruises are normal and everyone gets them. But they do signal that our body has become injured and sometimes there are limits to what they body can do all by itself.

If you feel your bruise is too large, or if the impact or trauma might have been too intense and might have caused other problems, then you may wish to seek medical attention.

Of course, everyone is different and everyone's health is also different. If you suffer from any diseases or medical condition that might make bruising more serious or dangerous, you should treat any bruise accordingly. If you have any doubts or concerns regarding whether or not any bruise is serious or a cause of concern, you should check with your doctor.

How Long Should it Take
for a Bruise to Go Away?

If a person is healthy and has no illnesses or health related diseases, most bruises will disappear within approx. 2 weeks. Now keep in mind that some bruises might take a little longer and some might disappear in less time. It all depends on the severity of the injury and other circumstances.

Usually the first five days or so the bruise will be purplish or black and blue. Over the next 5 to 10 days the bruise will gradually get lighter and turn into a green or yellowish color during that time. Finally, over the last 5-7 days the bruise will turn yellow and eventually get lighter until it is totally gone.

These time frames will vary from person to person and also on how well the bruise was treated, how the patient rested or protected the area and several other factors.

Medications and medical history and overall condition of health can also play an important role. Generally speaking the elderly might take longer because their bodies take longer to heal in general.

The location of the bruise may also play a significantly role in the length of time it will take for the bruise to disappear. Bruises on the bottoms of our feet might take longer because we cannot totally rest that area because life goes on and life usually requires a certain level of mobility.

The RICER Protocol

For those of you who are not aware of it, there is a specific protocol involved in the treatment of bruises. This protocol is called the R.I.C.E.R. protocol. R.I.C.E.R. stands for Rest, Ice, Compression, Elevation and Referral. These are the five most important basic steps in treating and controlling damage of bruising.

We are going to discuss each part of the RICER protocol in the upcoming pages but we want to stress now that this protocol is what should always be followed when it comes to bruising. These are the basics and the things that will give you the most benefit.

This is because RICER helps address the most important aspect of controlling the damage done by bruising. By following some simple steps and techniques we cannot only reduce the size and damage to the surrounding area but help aid the body in healing faster as well.

The result is less bruising initially and a more rapid reduction in the appearance of the bruised area as well.

RICER is a general purpose protocol to address various medical issues. But it is NOT a definitive approach that is good for all applications. At times there might be other factors which make applying one or more of the RICER components either impractical or ill-advised. If in doubt, please contact your doctor or other medical professional.

When to Seek Medical Attention

While we are not doctor's and while only doctors or trained medical professionals are the only ones who can make an accurate and safe diagnosis, there are a couple of things you should look for whenever you sustain an bruise or impact caused injury.

First of all, any impact that is immediately followed by a sharp or severe pain or the inability to use or place weight on the area is an indication of possibly a more serious condition and you should get that checked out. Bruises can be tender and the surrounding area can be sensitive and tender as well. But sharp or severe pain is usually suggestive of something else.

While bruise might swell slightly over time after the impact if there is immediate swelling or severe swelling, that is another indication that something more serious may be going on and that you should get a professional examination.

Also. After an impact you usually will not see bruising immediately afterwards. Full bruising may not be noticeable for several hours or possibly a day or two afterwards. If you experience an impact and see bruising immediately afterwards, I would seek a medical opinion as well. It is better to be safe than sorry.

Bruising on the head can be serious as well because of potential injury to the brain. If you or the patient had lost consciousness or cannot remember things, then you should seek medical attention to check for a concussion. If you have a headache after the impact that should be checked as well. In that case the bruise should be the least of your concerns.

If the bruise in on or near your face, it will usually appear worse just because of where it is. But, if it affects your vision or if it prevents you from making normal eye movements, seek medical attention.

If the bruise does not appear to be healing or going away within two weeks or is not totally gone within 3-4 weeks get it checked by your doctor.

If you are currently on any kind of blood thinning medication make your doctor aware of the bruising. Medical intervention might be required to start the normal healing process. This must be done in accordance with your doctor. Do NOT make any alterations to your meds without your doctor's approval.

What to Do First

This one might appear to be common sense but despite that people fail to do the most important thing when it comes to bruising. That is to immediately stop what you were doing that caused the bruising in the first place!

For example, if you slipped and fell because it was very icy outside, then you should go back inside and stay off the icy surfaces until it is safe and you have healed. If you were playing sports and were hit and injured, take yourself out of the game if the impact was severe or at the first sign of bruising if it appear significant.

A bruise is the body's way of telling you that it is damaged under the skin. You cannot see the vessels themselves but when you see a bruise, you know some of them were damaged in that area. So view the bruise as the body's way of telling you it helps some help.

Do not continue the activity that caused the problem in the first place. This is important because if an area becomes damaged in your body additional impacts or damage to that same area will result in even more damage. Your body has been weakened in areas and you need to protect your body.

So if you fell down the steps on the icy walk, going out again and falling a second time might cause you severe injuries. If you took a vicious hit on the basketball court, a second hit could result in even more damage. Of course, the more severe the damage the longer the recovery time.

Bruise Treatment Tips, Options & Techniques

Apply Ice to Constrict Blood Vessels

When an impact first occurs that you feel is significant to either cause swelling or bruising, the first step should be to ice the area as soon as possible. The cold helps constrict the blood vessels and this helps reduce the amount of blood that seeps into area surrounding the injury. So the less blood that enters the area the smaller the bruise.

The best practice is to apply ice wrapped in a cloth bag or towel and apply it to the affected area for roughly 15 minutes. Then remove the ice and allow the skin to come back to room temperature naturally. Continue this practice for as long as you feel necessary. If you see minor swelling, continue the ice therapy. Of course, if you see major swelling, you should go for medical treatment or evaluation.

Always wrap the ice in a towel or cloth. This helps protect the skin from the extremely low temperature of the ice. Frostbite and other damage can occur if ice comes into direct contact with the skin of significant period of time.

One effective and handy option is to use a bag of frozen vegetables such as peas as a source of cold. The peas are small and will more readily move to form against the entire area to provide uniform cooling. Depending on the size of ice cubes, you might have small areas of your skin that are not exposed to any of the cooling.

Naturally if the fall, impact, or trauma has pierced or cut the skin, that should be addressed immediately and ice applied after wards once the skin has been repaired and sealed.

Apply Compression

Depending on the location of the bruise, you should consider applying some form of compression to the area. That means using some kind of compression bandage wrapped around the area to help control swelling.

Using an elastic bandage wrapped around the area will help control the swelling by helping to move fluids out of the area. But take care to wrap the bandage properly. If you warp it too tight you can inhibit proper blood flow in that area of the body.

This can cause serious problems if a too tight bandage is left in place for too long. If you wrap the bandage too tight you may experience tingling, coolness, pain and swelling below the bandage. If you experience any of these symptoms, or if you just feel the bandage is too tight, loosen it. If someone else is applying the bandage for you, let them know when you think it is too tight.

Usually wrapping is necessary for the first 24 to maybe 48 hours. If you think you need to use compression for longer periods than 48 hours you should consult a medical professional so that more serious conditions can be ruled out or confirmed. Failure to do this may cause serious repercussions.

After the First day, Apply Heat

After the first 24 hours or so, you can apply gentle warm heat to the area to dilate the blood vessels and help promote the natural healing process. This will allow the body to naturally break down the blood in the bruise and remove it naturally from the affected area.

Keep the heat levels lower so as to not overheat the skin. You can use hot towels, hot water bottles or other forms of heat.

A heating pad could also be used but take care not to use the hotter settings. We want to stimulate the area we want to heal not burn it.

Elevate the area

When blood vessels have broken in an area, the blood pools in that area resulting in the bruising. If we elevate the area we reduce the amount of pooling as blood spreads out further to surrounding areas. The body is then able to remove it faster and easier and swelling is reduced as well. Both reducing swelling and being able to remove blood through the natural healing process both result in smaller and faster healing bruises.

You can elevate legs and arms by placing a pillow under them. Other areas of the body might be a little more difficult. If you bruise a hip or thigh, you can sleep on the good side so the bruised area is higher. Just make sure to just elevate it slightly and not so high that you develop tingling or numbness on any part of your body.

When it comes to elevation, try to elevate the bruised area above your heart. This will help drain fluids and blood back to the heart.

Rest the Area

Remember that a bruise represents damage to the blood vessels in a certain area.

So this area has sustained an injury even if the area is not painful. Therefore it makes sense that if any area of your body becomes injured we should rest that area and not involve it in any kind of strenuous activity.

That means if you bruise your arms, you should not go to the gym and lift weights. If you bruise your hip you wouldn't go on the treadmill. Any kind of strenuous activity will place a strain on the area and possibly cause a re-injury of the recently healed blood vessels.

The idea is to stop most activity when you are first injured and when gradually increase the level of activity as you heal. Eventually you will get back to normal exercise and activity levels after the area has healed and the bruise has disappeared.

Gently Massage the Area

After the first day, gently massaging the bruised area several times a day can help assist the body's naturally healing process.

It would also help flush the toxins and internal debris away from the area. This should be done as long as the area is not painful. If the area is extremely tender or painful then hold off until the area stabilizes and is no longer painful.

Use pressure on the area sufficient to adequately help the body but not to the point where it becomes painful. If massaging is painful then you may be doing it too hard and you should use lighter pressure. Over time as the area heals you might be able to use slightly higher pressure but remember this process should be soothing to the area and not harsh.

For some people, using a licensed massage therapist or physical therapist to perform the massage might be preferable. This is especially true for areas that you might not be able to reach comfortably by yourself. Plus, an experienced person will know how hard to press, how long to massage and the proper way to massage the area to get the best benefits.

Expose it to Sunlight

If possible, exposing the bruised area to sunlight can help the body break down the substances under the skin and facilitate healing. Sunlight contains ultraviolet light which helps break down bilirubin which causes the yellowish look of the bruise as it heals.

You don't need copious amounts of sun to accomplish this. Sometimes just 10 to 15 minutes a day of sunlight will be all that you need to help the body and the healing process. Any longer and you might get the area sunburned which will cause additional problems to an already injured area. Because of this, use sunscreen when required to protect the top of the skin as the area underneath is healing.

It has also been said that natural sunlight is good for the entire body in general so any time you can get in the sun, as long as it is not too much, will help not only heal the bruise but help your entire immune system.

Avoid Alcohol

Since alcohol is known to act like a blood thinner, stay away from it during the healing process. This will help minimize the internal bleeding by speeding up the healing process. Alcohol can also decrease the levels of vitamin C in the body which will inhibit the healing process.

Not only that but people under the influence of alcohol will often have their balance and other senses diminished. This increases the likelihood of bumping into things and falling during the healing process

. For this reason, and to further protect the area throughout the healing process, stay away from alcohol until the healing process has been completed.

By the way, if the reason for the impact or bruising was a fall caused by alcohol in the first place then you should deal with what might be an alcohol abuse problem. Failure to address the root cause of any problem will not allow you to make the much needed changes and choices in the future.

Bruising Pain Relief

If the bruise is accompanied by pain or tenderness due to the impact, consider taking acetaminophen to relieve the pain. Try and stay away from aspirin as it acts like a blood thinner and will affect the ability of the blood to clot properly. Check with your doctor if you have concerns about which is the best pain relief option for you.

Sometimes using heat will alleviate pain as well. Take pain medications of the proper type if needed but do not take them when they are no longer necessary. Remember that pain and soreness are the body's way of telling you an area needs rest or attention. So pain is not always bad. But if the pain is affecting your movements or quality of life, take the appropriate medications.

Take Some Vitamin C

Vitamin C deficiency can cause easy bruising and more severe bruising. Vitamin C helps protect the area around our blood vessels and without this protective layer, or when this protective layer is thinner or weaker than usual, bruising can be easier and more profound. Vitamin C also helps builds collagen which promotes healing of the skin.

This is not a case of too much is always better. When it comes to putting any supplement or medication in your system, do so only with the approval of your doctor. Too much of any vitamin might not be a good thing so if you are not sure if your vitamin levels are low, consult with your doctor. Simple blood tests can check for the levels of several vitamins and other factors that might contribute to or effect bruising.

Gravity & Bruising

If you have a bruise on your face or legs, you might notice that the bruise travels or migrates lower over the course of the first few days.

This is because as the blood enters the area gravity acts upon it and this causes the blood to flow lower.

Bruises around the eyes will more rapidly move lower and bruises on the thighs and legs will tend to do the same. The upper arms may do so as well. Lower arm bruises, which sometimes might not be lower might migrate less.

There is little that you can do to stop this other than laying down so gravity will not be as strong. But that is not practical as few people are capable or able to stay in e reclined position for one or two weeks. If you have a bruise that is not exposed when it first starts, lying down as much as possible may help keep it from becoming exposed over time. But be aware that there is usually settling or lowering all almost all larger bruises. The more blood under the skin, the larger role gravity will play in the healing process.

Bruising Under Nails

When trauma or impact comes on a nail, the result might be a bruise under the nail. This usually requires a different type of treatment if the bruise cannot drain.

If the bruise is under the skin which is under the nail, then you might be fine. But if the bruise you see is from blood which has entered the space between the nail and the skin that could cause you trouble.

Blood that gets in between the skin and the nail acts like a balloon that tries to force the nail away from the skin. As the heart pumps, the blood is pushed into the space and pressure is exerted on the nail. This can create a large amount of pain which sometimes can be throbbing in nature.

If the nail is a toe nail then it might be painful for someone to walk or step with the foot that has the problem. If the damage is on a fingernail, the person might have a problem gripping something, holding a pen or other device or even moving the finger.

When this happens, sometimes soaking the toe or finger in warm water will soften the nail and allow the blood to drain out naturally. Eventually the pressure will force the blood out if the nail / skin barrier is small.

You might try to GENTLY lift the nail up SLIGHTLY to help things along a bit. But be careful. If you feel more pain, then stop and continue soaking or seek medical attention.

If that doesn't work, you might have to go to the doctor who will drill a small hole into the nail to drain the blood and remove the pressure.

This is done with a sterile drill so DO NOT try this at home! Have it done by a doctor or ER professional only.

Apply Arnica Ointment

This ointment or gel is well known to dilate blood vessels and reduce blood seepage into the area of the bruise. This will minimize the size and depth of the bruise.

Arnica is also available in pill form as well. Taken as directed this can ease the discomfort of sore muscles while also promoting the healing process when it comes to bruises. It is available over the counter

Eat Pineapple or

Take a Supplement

Pineapple contains Bromelain which is an enzyme known to reduce bruising.

This enzyme is available in a supplement that can be taken to dissolve blood clots and fade bruises. You should use this enzyme only after doctor approval as it can interact with your other medications and supplements.

Pineapples also contain vitamin C which is known to bolster the healing process when available in sufficient quantities.

Blood Thinners & Bruising

For certain medical conditions, some people might be on aspirin or prescription blood thinners. When a person is on blood thinners they bleed more and for longer periods of time before the blood clots properly. That means bleeding will continue longer so more blood will be released into the area surrounding the impact.

This means bruising will be easier, larger and more severe. This might not mean anything else in the body is wrong but rather it is just the blood thinners doing their job. Since blood thinners are designed to stop the body from created blood clots which can cause serious problems, it just makes sense that they will affect normal clotting as well.

If you are on blood thinners, please address bruising with your doctor to make sure you are on the correct dosage and are not in fact taking too higher a dose. Do NOT make this decision by yourself. Consult your doctor, have the required tests and then make a medically sound decision after you have all the information.

Light Activity after 72 Hours

Some people think that you should rest after sustaining a significant bruise and they are 100% correct.

Resting allows the area of the bruise to heal and recover. But after 72 hours it is desirable to return to LIGHT activity.

Light activity helps stimulate the area which promotes healing and the flushing of toxins and blood from the area surrounding the injury site. But we stress the "light" part of the process. If you have a bruise on your thigh then you can walk a little to stimulate the area. But you should not run 10 miles at full speed as that can do more damage than good.

Like everything else in life, ease back into things in moderation. If you start to feel pain or discomfort then dial things back a little bit. You can do a little bit more as the bruise fades but remember that even though the tenderness and stiffness might have gone away the area is still healing and should not be placed under strain.

Diet & Health & Bruising

If you are someone who bruises easily or for no apparent reason, you may want to consider going to the doctor and making them aware of this.

Bruising without a legitimate reason might be a symptom of other issues going on within your body.

Your diet can also play a significant role in bruising as well. Foods that are very high in vitamin K help promote clotting but can also interact with anti-coagulants prescribed for heart disease and other disorders. Vitamin C deficiencies can also lead to clotting issues as well.

If you think that your diet may be causing or contributing to bruising or clotting issues, see your doctor so that they can do the necessary blood tests or other test they deem necessary. They can also go through your medical history and issues and use the test results plus your individual history to come up with an appropriate diet.

A well balanced diet will not only help your bruises heal better and faster but will also help you live longer and healthier at the same time. So even if you do not have a bruising problem, eat healthier just because it is the right thing to do.

Bruising of the Heel

When we get a bruise on the bottom of the heel that can be a difficult thing to treat effectively. You should stay off your feet to avoid reinjuring the area and you might even have to take weight of the heel when you walk if the injury is severe enough.

When you get a heel bruise, the best course of action is to use the RICER protocol and use rest, ice, compression, elevation and refer to a medical expert for proper treatment if necessary. You should not ignore a heel bruise as continuing the same activity which caused the bruise will just make things worse.

You should try your best to not walk on the heel until it is pain free to do so. Remember that pain is the boy's way of telling us that healing needs to take place. If you must walk, limit the walking to the bare minimum. Use a cane or crutches to remove as much of the weight from the heel as possible.

Be careful though because if you walk with a different gait or form you can place stress on other joints and bones in the body. This can cause other problems in the body as well as increasing the likelihood of falling, tripping and other similar problems.

The best approach for heel bruises should be on prevention.

This means wearing high quality footwear that is properly sized for your feet. If the activity is especially hard on the bottom of the feet such as long distance running or climbing then you may wish to wear a protective heel cover to provide additional protection to the heel. Another possibility is to use some shock absorbing insoles to help absorb some of the shock to the bottom of your feet during running or exercise.

Heel injuries are easier to get if you are walking or exercising without footwear especially when walking on uneven surfaces. Your feet are routinely subjected to a lot of abuse and you should take whatever steps you can to minimize the stress and damage to them. This is a necessity if you have to walk over hard and jagged surfaces. Stepping on a sharp rock with the bottom of your feet can cause bruising and possibly more serious issues.

Bruised Ribs

If you receive a blow or impact in the rib area, you might push the ribs into the surrounding muscles and tissues and cause a rib bruise. Rib bruises can be very painful and even debilitating when they occur.

This is because as we move and breathe, our ribs move against the injured tissue. Sneezing and coughing can be uncomfortable or even very painful. If you have ever bruised a rib, you know what we are talking about.

If you have very severe pain there might be a possibility that you have actually broken a rib. If the blow or impact was severe enough to cause that type of injury then perhaps it might be a good idea to get checked by your doctor or take a trip to the ER. Left untreated a broken rib could puncture a lung which can be very serious.

Bruised ribs respond well to the RICER protocol. Because of the almost constant movement of the ribs bruising in this area can take a bit loner to fully heal. 3-4 weeks is not uncommon when it comes to rib bruises.

When it comes to rib bruises, immediately stopping any activity which has the potential to cause further injury to the rib area is critical. The ribs protect vital areas of our body and we must take the utmost care when injuries to this area are incurred.

As far as recovery is concerned, stay away from any activity that involves the rib area and the muscles around it. Even cardio work can be bad because any kind of exercise makes you breathe faster and every time we breathe the ribs move. Wait at least 3-4 weeks to resume normal physical activity and even then, the area should be pain free.

You may wish to consider wearing protective gear in the future when performing similar activities. This will help you avoid, or at least minimize, injuries to the ribs in the future. Once you experience a rib injury, you would want to do your best to avoid them in the future.

Leave the Skin Intact

Most of the time a bruise will just be a bruise and the skin will not be broken.

If that is the case then we just need to deal with minimizing the blood seepage and get the healing process started. But sometimes an impact will cause the skin to become cut, broken or you might suffer an abrasion as well.

Any break in the skin exposes the body to infection and other issues. If to skin is broken, wash and clean it according to establish medical practices and apply an anti-biotic ointment. Then keep the area clean by covering it with a bandage of some type to protect and shield the area.

Naturally if the break in the skin is larger or bleeding heavily, that should be your primary concern and you should get that checked as quickly as possible. Deep or very wide cuts should be attended to by trained medical professionals.

If the skin is not actually cut but you have suffered an abrasion, clean the area to remove any dirt or foreign matter and then apply the ointment and apply a bandage. Just because the skins is not physically open does not mean infection cannot occur. If the skin is abraded and raw, protect it with a bandage.

Always remember that our skin is the primary barrier between the insides of our bodies and everything that is in our environment. Take care of it and protect it. This will help our skin stay healthy, flexible and less prone to bruising.

Your Meds & Bruising

Depending on your health and medical conditions, you might be taking medications that can either make you more prone to bruising and also making bruising more seriously when it does occur. Medications such as anti-inflammatories, sometimes anti-depressants and other medications can affect clotting in some fashion.

People who take medications for heart disease should be especially careful as some of these medications are blood thinners designed to make clotting more difficult. The more of these meds that you are on, the less your body will clot when it is injured. So minor problems can result in major bruising.

If you bruise easily, or if bruises appear to be larger or more intense than they should be, you should consult your doctor and talk to him about it. While there may not be anything that you can do about it, just being aware about your health and medicine's role in bruising might cause you to be more careful or react faster when you experience any impact that might result in a bruise.

Sex, Aging & Bruising

As people get older, their skin undergoes subtle changes. This happens because there is less fat under the skin and this results in less cushioning. So even a lesser impact on an older person might result in considerable bruising.

While there is no cure for this happening as we get older, eating right and staying healthy will not only help protect our bodies but will also help keep us from easily bruising and minimizing the impact when we do.

Older adults, for many reasons, might be more susceptible to falls which usually result in bruising as well. In those cases, care should be taken to make the environment easier to navigate for the older people.

For some reason, woman often bruise easier than men especially around the areas of the buttocks, thighs and underarms. This has to do with the different body composition between men and women.

Healing Bruises in Children

Children all gets bumps and bruises. After all, they are young, they are inquisitive and they do not have the experience or sometimes common sense to not do certain things that might have a slightly dangerous side.

So it is not a case of when a child gets a bruise it is going to be when and how bad the bruise is.

What is different, though, is how we approach bruises in order to help the child understand what is happening and not be scared or afraid of that dark blue or black area that somehow is on their arm or leg right now.

When an adult gets a bruise, we know what's going on. We usually expect it after getting hit or taking a fall. We understand that a bruise is the usual result. So there is no fear or even concern or shock. We experience a trauma we expect a bruise and we deal with it.

But when a child gets a bruise, especially a deep or large bruise, they might be scared when they see the result.

So the parent or adult that is there when it happens should explain what is happening and let them know it is normal for the body to bruise when it gets hit and that the bruise will gradually get lighter and then go away. This way the child will not be afraid or scared about the changes they see on their skin.

Another difference is that when an adult gets injured most of us have the knowledge and common sense to know that we need to take it easy for the next week or two.

But a child, who usually goes through life at full speed all the time, might not do that. So we need to make sure the child is aware of the need to rest and then monitor their activity to make sure that they really do rest and are not running around like little tornadoes.

Children also tend to have a lower tolerance of pain than adults do. So the parent or supervising adult should make every effort to comfort the child and make the child comfortable.

The manner in which these objectives are accomplished should be left up to the parent or supervising adult.

Prevention and Pro-Active Care

Now that we know how to best care for bruising when it occurs, it just makes sense to understand that the best course of action is to create a lifestyle aimed at preventing bruises.

In other words, concentrate on doing things that will help you avoid the bruises in the first place so you don't have to treat them in the first place.

Since overall health and the ability for blood to clot properly is very important when it comes to bruising, it is important to have a healthy diet with adequate amounts of all vitamins and minerals. Be sure to include vegetables, whole grains and sources of protein as well. Deficiencies of vitamins K, C or B12 or folic acid can cause affect the ability of the blood to clot.

If you are bruising far too easily or if light impacts cause large bruising, you may have a problem with blood clotting. Check with your doctor if you experience this. They can do blood tests to see if you are taking supplements or medications that might affect blood clotting.

As we have already stated, anti-inflammatories, anti-coagulants and aspirin are known to change the way our blood clots. For most of us this will not create many problems. But for some of us, this may lead to an increase of bruising.

But the overall positive benefits of the medicines in other areas make them good choices for us. Only our doctors can properly advise us as to what the proper course of action should be.

Another area of concern just might be in your environment. If your bruises are caused by constantly tripping or bumping into things, consider removing clutter or objects you routinely come in contact with. Clutter is one of the most common causes of trips and falls.

If you know you are going to be involved in any activity or action that will likely involve physical contact, strongly consider wearing the appropriate safety or protection equipment. This equipment will protect important areas of your body from far more than just bruising. They will help keep you free of injury and bruising as well.

Bruising on Others

It would not be responsible to have a publication on treating and prevention of bruising without mentioning abuse. Bruising is one of the most visible and easily identifying things when it comes to discovering abuse. If you know of someone who frequently has bruising on any part of their body, they could be the victim of abuse.

If you suspect abuse, report it to the local authorities, abuse hotline or local health professional. Sometimes the victims are too afraid to talk to anyone about it because they are afraid of the repercussions for doing so. You might be their only friend or ally.

As we have already mentioned, the elderly and young children are more prone to bruising because of their lifestyle and physical limitations. So they might experience bruising more often than you or I. But if a pattern of bruising should appear over time this should be checked out to make sure that abuse or certain medical conditions are not causing the bruising.

Bruising After Surgical Procedures.

Any kind of surgical procedure where the skin is broken of the area is penetrated or cut in any way will induce bleeding and in most cases some swelling. Depending on the location of the surgery and the amount of work performed, the bruising or trauma may be minor or quite severe.

But when it comes to surgery and bruising, do not follow any of the instructions in this book or that you read online. Surgery involves far more than just a bruise. There was work done in your body that requires special care, treatment and rehabilitation.

Because of this, you should follow your doctor's instructions as far as icing, heat, washing and other types of treatment.

Follow your doctors rehab schedule, go to your follow-up appointments and do not stray from that regimen. If you do, you risk making the area worse, cause problems with proper healing and possibly suffer set-backs in your overall rehabilitation.

Bruising Without Apparent Reason

Sometimes we will notice a bruise and wonder why we have it in the first place. If we do not remember any kind of blow, impact or trauma, then something else may be going on that we are not aware of.

Anytime we have a bruise it is because we have had a blood vessel or something break or open to drain blood into the area. The bruise is merely a visual indication that something is wrong or not as it should be.

If you find a bruise on your body and you do not know how it got there, you may want to get it checked by your doctor. Especially if there is a lump or pain in the same area. Sometimes this is easy to spot depending on the area.

But if the bruise in in the groin or other area, you should get it checked out. It is far better to find out now that it was nothing than to let it go and have it turned into a major issue.

Bruising Myths

Try these if you want, or if your doctor suggests, but these are considered to be just old wives tales:

Placing a steak on a bruise will not help heal it or reduce it in size or intensity. You will just ruin a good steak unless you eat it right afterwards! The only positive thing that might happen is that if the steak was cold enough, it could be a source of cold which will help reduce swelling. But ice would do the same thing more efficiently and at a far lower cost!

Baking soda is not a treatment for bruises either. Though taking a bath can relieve muscle soreness, it is not an effective treatment for bruises. While it can't really hurt, it won't help either.

Rubbing a hard-boiled egg over the bruise to enhance circulation has nothing to do with the hard-boiled egg itself. If any benefit is achieved it was because of the massaging nature of the rubbing not the egg. So use =light massage when it is safe and leave the egg in the fridge!

Preparation H might numb the area around the bruise and might reduce swelling slightly but it will not help make the bruise go away faster to otherwise help the healing process.

Conclusion

Most bruises are just a nuisance and a part of our daily lives. We all get them and we all have to deal with them. But no matter how insignificant they might seem we need to take them seriously. Hopefully after reading this book you have become a little bit more aware with what bruises are and how to properly treat them. You also know what to do and what decisions to make when you sustain a bruise.

Once again, please consult your doctor when it comes to making any medical decisions and do not make this book a substitute or alternative for getting proper medical care and evaluation.

Also Available from 26Ways.com:

26 Ways to Get More Fun from
RC Aircraft

26 Ways to Save Money on
Your Utility Bills

26 Ways to Manage Your
Type 2 Diabetes & Control
Your Blood sugar

26 Ways to Become
A Better Manager

26 Ways to Grow Your
On-Line Business

26 Ways to Be the Best Wife Ever!

For all other Publications,
and for more information on our
books and manuals, please visit our
website at:

http://www.26ways.com

www.ingramcontent.com/pod-product-compliance
Lightning Source LLC
Chambersburg PA
CBHW071145280526
45787CB00003B/1415